1

The Reservoir of Better Health

Small Changes, Done Consistently...

Charles F. Roost, D.C.

2nd Edition

INTRODUCTION

Have you ever seen how healthy a new born baby looks? The supple, full, rosy, resilient look of them? One of the reasons for this vibrant appearance is the fact that they are born with a full **Reservoir of Health**. Have you witnessed the endless energy and exuberance of a three year old during play time? Again, the child's Reservoir is full of what they need to function at 100% of their potential. This Reservoir holds the sum total of all of the good 'stuff' we each need in order to deal with the stresses of life – and at birth, that reservoir is chock full. The Reservoir of Health is a depository of important physical, emotional and spiritual stuff like proteins, vitamins, hormones, enzymes and minerals, as well as less tangible resources such as purpose, love and hope.

A full Reservoir allows us to flourish with the ability to draw from this critical pool of resources to deal with life's demands. It gives us the ability to grow, fight off viruses, and heal broken bones, as well as the amazing capacity to respond to car problems, time crunches, difficult relationships and other stresses. It provides the resources that allow us to respond to opportunities and to create new and beautiful aspects of life. Unfortunately, responding to these ubiquitous needs and opportunities gradually drains the Reservoir, leaving less and less resources available for the next crisis.

As the Reservoir empties, we find ourselves showing signs that should tell us that something is wrong. Take a moment and evaluate your current life experience. See if you experience any of these warning signs:

3

- decreased energy
- slower healing
- lowered productivity
- more frequent illnesses
- poor sleep
- lessening creativity
- lack of former levels of creativity
- mood swings
- deteriorating relationships

Typically these issues do not show up until our third or fourth decade of life, but in our stress-overloaded culture, they are being experienced by people as early as their second decade of life and even younger. Often when we experience these issues, we explain to ourselves, (and to anyone else who will listen), that our health issues are due to 'getting older', accrued old injuries, or even genetic issues. But buying into these false explanations for our declining health condemns us unnecessarily to poor health. Don't allow these common excuses to distract you from the real possibility of finding better health.

But just what is 'health'? Most of us fall into the easy habit of defining our health by how good we feel. A lack of symptoms must mean that we are healthy – right? Well – not exactly. There are actually three parts to truly being well. Three aspects to being fully healthy. Each of the three are important. Each of the three impacts the others. Each is measurable. But none of the three is totally objective. The quality of each varies wildly under the impact of dozens of factors ranging from mood, to weather, to stress levels, to how busy we are. One of the frustrating things about this concept is that the most obvious of the three factors is arguably the least important one.

4

The three factors that, added together, determine how healthy we are?

- How we **feel** – symptoms
- How we **function** – How well can I do what I want to do without paying for it later in pain and stiffness
- **Degenerative** issues – underlying, often 'silent' issues that we may not notice until years into the process when it is much more difficult to fix

This is the **Rule of Three**. Three components of our health. Added together, they total how close we live to 100% of our potential.

Now, obviously, the symptom factor is the one that gets most of our attention. Pain will get our attention. But symptoms are tricky – we can feel uncomfortable either when we have a big health issue (a broken bone, a serious disease process) or when our body is reacting in a healthy way in fighting off a problem (a fever, vomiting to rid the stomach of a toxin). Symptoms matter, but can fool us into thinking we are well when we aren't, or thinking we are in trouble when our bodies are functioning normally.

Function will actually tell us more accurately about how healthy we are. If we feel pretty healthy, yet avoid doing activities that we need to do, or love to do, because if we do them we will pay for it later in pain and stiffness – we are not healthy. That is not functioning at 100%. That is not healthy. Restrictions in our activities of daily living is a significant indication of how healthy we are – or how far from it we are.

Degenerative issues can include joint conditions (arthritis), muscle issues (fibro-myalgia), or chemical problems (diabetes). Each of these start quietly, but cascade into debilitating, life-destroying factors. These are critical factors

5

in any attempt to evaluate how healthy we are. And if these factors can be detected and stopped early in their processes, we will be far healthier than attempting to catch and fix them years into the disease with all the momentum that comes with them.

Symptoms, Function and Degeneration – three prongs of the triad of health – the Rule of Three. Ignoring any one of them will result in less than the function we were designed to enjoy. The good news is that there is hope! There is a system of health and wellness that will maximize symptoms, maximize function, and interrupt degeneration. That system lies in understanding and investing in your Reservoir of Health.

Fortunately, just as the Reservoir of Health is drained by the demands of life, it can also be refilled by pouring the right resources back into it. Simply put, there are six resources that will refill the Reservoir. Some are obvious. Others are more subtle, but still every bit as important. All of them can be addressed by making small changes in our lifestyle, and in our thinking.

The six essential building blocks of health that need to be consistently maintained to keep the Reservoir full are:

- **Bioavailable Nutrition** – this goes beyond eating three square meals a day
- **Quality Rest** – our minds and bodies heal and rebuild during proper sleep
- **Balanced Exercise** – balance means symmetry of motion in 5 areas of activity
- **Meaningful Stress Management** – there are practical ways to decrease the stress load, and to manage the impact of both chronic and acute stress

- **Practical Spiritual Health** – all of these factors impact one another, and this one is perhaps more important than any of the others
- **Neural Integrity** – there is one system that coordinates everything our bodies do, and it needs maintenance, too.

In this book we will explore how to make small, consistent changes in each of these areas that will return you to levels of health you have longed for, and perhaps given up hoping for, for years.

Three key aspects of health. Six basic ingredients to refilling the Reservoir of Health. Awareness of these concepts, and simple steps to maintain them, will result in each of us finding, fulfilling, and maximizing our purpose in life. Are you ready to invest in your health? Are you prepared to put in a little work in order to gain a better life?

Welcome! This book is one of the key means by which we, at Delta Health and Wellness try to give you, our client, tools to find improved health. Better health is available to every single person on this planet, and it is our mission to help people experience it.

Some of the tools you will learn in this book cost nothing more than time and determination. Others have some financial expense attached to them. But every one of the tools you will learn from this book is worth whatever it costs in time, effort, self-discipline, and finances. In a word, these recommendations work.

Some of the other means by which we offer these insights include DVDs about our methods, pamphlets and articles which we have available, and public presentations. Dr. Roost is available to speak to your group on topics including health, improving your energy, and productivity. If you are interested in arranging one of these presentations, please let our office know.

Delta Chiropractic Center has a few non-negotiable stances that you might want to be aware of. We believe that every person can improve their health. We believe that people are more than walking, talking assemblage of bone and muscle. In truth, we are complex beings made up of spirit, emotions, and mind, as well as body. Each of these facets must be addressed in order to maximize our health.

And finally, we believe that you are worth investing in. That is why we are here. That is what we have invested the last 33 years of our lives in. And we hope you will find this journey, our office, and this book to be well-fitted portions of that investment.

This book is a practical, applicable book, and deals with how you can find better health, just like thousands of other patients have who have come through our office since 1980. I hope that in reading this short book, you will be assisted in your journey toward better health, physically, emotionally, and spiritually.

Let's dig in!

Dr. Roost has been in private practice since 1980. He graduated Magna Cum Laude from Palmer College of Chiropractic, has served on state and national boards, and founded the Michigan Christian Chiropractors Association. He speaks on health topics such as maximizing energy, attaining goals, and stress management, and is the author of three other books.

Reservoir of Better Health

By Charles F. Roost, D.C.

Delta Chiropractic Center
722 N. Creyts Rd.
Lansing, MI 48917
www.Delta-Chiro.com

The Reservoir of Better Health

Small Changes, Done Consistently...

Contents

13

The Reservoir of Better Health
Small Changes, Done Consistently...

CHAPTER ONE

Wellness and the Reservoir of Health

It is amazing how much resilience our bodies hold. We can take incredible amounts of stress, trauma and environmental toxins, and can ignore the upkeep of our bodies for years, and still continue functioning very well. As young adults we can participate in contact sports, eat junk food, and sleep far less than we should - and still run at full speed all day long. For most of us it is not until we enter our 3rd, 4th, or even 5th decade of life that we begin noticing the impact of that kind of lifestyle. When it happens, though, it is as though we have drained **a reservoir of vitality**, and it is now all we can do to continue living a productive life.

Our health is maintained by a reservoir of resources from which we can draw to keep our health intact. It is apparent that we are born with a certain depository of resources – a reservoir filled up by our mothers before we are born. This reservoir is a bit like buying a car with a full tank of gas. We can drive it for a time, but if we fail to refill it, eventually it will go dry.

> **Technical Side Note** – the reservoir is made up of things like vitamin storage in our tissues, redundancy in nerve, muscle and soft tissue function, and the ability of our bodies to store a certain level of toxins safely before they "overflow the storage system" and cause noticeable problems.

Two other factors can shed light on this analogy, as well. First, there are a lot of activities we engage in that drain the

14

reservoir: eating fast foods, drinking soda pop, poor posture, ignoring the health of our spine until we have pain, abusing medications, alcohol or other drugs, lack of sound sleep, loneliness, ignoring the importance of our spiritual life, watching too much TV, filling our minds with negative inputs day after day, exposure to stress, bacteria and viruses, and generally ignoring health-maintenance concepts – all of these deplete the reservoir. On top of that, there are two other factors that work at draining the reservoir no matter what we do. No I'm not referring to our in-laws. I'm speaking of time and gravity. These unstoppable facts of life constantly wear on us, and force us to slowly use resources from our Reservoir of Health.

The good news is that there are things we can do to replenish this reservoir. Eating healthy food, drinking uncontaminated water, taking quality vitamins, engaging in regular exercise, getting proper sleep, practicing good posture, getting regular spinal checkups, purposefully inputting positive materials into our minds, managing our stress levels, pursuing spiritual health, and having healthy friendships are examples of activities that refill the storage tank of our health. In fact, there are six basic areas to which we must pay attention in order to fill the reservoir, and in order to function at 100%:

- **Nutrition**
- **Rest**
- **Exercise**
- **Spinal Function**
- **Stress Management**
- **The Spiritual Component**

Most people can get away with ignoring these six essential ingredients to health for years, because we have a reservoir that we can tap into – for awhile. Remember how indestructible you felt as a teenager? Remember knowing that you couldn't be hurt? Remember feeling that, statistics aside, it wouldn't happen to me? Eventually, however, we find ourselves with a health problem, and wonder two things:

1) **What did we do to get there?**
2) **Why is it so hard to get better?**

The answer to both of these questions lies in the nature of the Reservoir of Health. While there may not have been anything obvious that caused our latest descent into sickness or pain, there usually is a pattern of draining the reservoir, or failing to replenish one or more of the six basic resources, that allowed us to gradually become more susceptible to sickness and more unhealthy.

On the other hand, once we start having symptoms, or other health issues, we regain enough motivation to begin replenishing those resources. We start eating better, getting spinal care, exercising and taking vitamins, and we gradually refill the reservoir. Unfortunately, symptoms rarely disappear as soon as we start refilling. There seems to be a level of resources in the reservoir to which we must refill and maintain before the body has time and proper materials to begin healing, and only then do the symptoms start to subside.

This can be frustrating, because we know we are doing the right things, yet we are still not feeling better. My advice is to be patient, continue doing the right things, and eventually these amazing organisms called our bodies, can and will heal themselves from a wide array of diseases and malfunctions. This is the **Law of Health** that states that "if we get rid of interference, and give our bodies what they need – we will heal."

16

Finally, it is critical to know that wellness – the ability to function at 100% of our capacity – is more than feeling symptom free. It is critical to go on filling the reservoir with ingredients from each of the six basic building blocks every day. Even when we are feeling well, we must pay attention to restoring the resources, the stockpile, the Reservoir of Health, against the day when the stresses of life hit us hard. We must be ready to fight back with those resources. If we wait to do the right things until stresses strike, it is too late. We will end up paying a higher price than we had to.

Waiting to deal with our health until we have symptoms is much like waiting to file our tax return until the IRS calls. It is too late. The damage is already done, and we will now pay a bigger price than we needed to initially.

It's important to note that most of the things that we do in the six basic areas of health to refill the reservoir are not necessarily very fun, nor do they necessarily cause an immediate, noticeably good feeling with which to reward our good behavior. However, they are still important to do.

I don't feel better after I swallow my vitamins, but I know that good, quality vitamins are doing their part in refilling my health reservoir with resources that will keep me healthier longer. I'd rather spend my money on a book than on a bottle of vitamins, but I buy the vitamins anyway.

Often, I find myself thinking that I'd rather go to a movie than run and lift weights. But I work out anyway – usually 5 times each week – because I know that if I don't, I'll pay a harsher price later for taking the easy way.

I may not have back pain to remind me to get my spine adjusted, and to feel immediate relief from afterward, yet I know that keeping my nerves free of interference will make me more able to resist strains and traumas that can decimate my health. I do these things, not so that I will merely feel better, but because I want to stay healthy, resist diseases, and hold up well under stresses.

CHAPTER 2

The Reservoir of Health – The Six, Slick, Super-Essential Building Blocks to Better Health

If health is a building, you must install 6 foundational blocks – six corner stones to the edifice – if you want the building to stand in a storm. If health is a jigsaw puzzle, there are six crucial pieces that bring clarity to the completed picture. If health is a stool, there are six irreplaceable legs that are necessary to build a piece of furniture stabile enough to sit on. If health is a cake, there are six essential ingredients to combine for it to come out properly. If health is going to last through the stresses that life brings, if it is going to keep you going as the years pass, if you want to maintain a level of function as time passes, and wear and tear add up, then you must work on all six of these critical aspects of health.

Ingredients. Just how important are they? Can't I bake a cake if I'm only leaving out one or two items on the list? Let's explore that idea. No eggs? No problem. Bake it and see what comes out. Short on some shortening? Don't bother the neighbors. Just mix up what you've got and taste the results.

Perhaps not. It is obvious that each ingredient really does have an important part to play in the final product. And while a cake is a small thing to risk experimentation on, our health is not. What we do with our Reservoir of Health matters. How diligent we are in replacing the six essential building blocks makes a big difference. Again, we can ignore this information for a long time, and still function pretty well. Unfortunately, by the time we've gone through ten or fifteen or twenty years mixing only most and not all of the ingredients, we have accumulated damage, and it's too late. With that much abuse of the system done, it is much, much harder to go back.

On the bright side, however, I am convinced that it is never too late to make a change, to take a step up, and to improve on your health from where it currently is. The Law of Health stands ready to step in and act on our behalf, if we just play by the rules that govern that law.

Ingredients matter. And the ingredients for health and a fully balanced life include:

- Nutrition
- Rest
- Exercise
- Spinal function
- Stress Management
- Spiritual wellness

Mix them all wisely, and you will add years to your health, and health to your years. Leave any one of them out, and sooner or later, you will have to pay the price.

We at the Delta Health and Wellness offer help with each of these ingredients. Please take the time to evaluate each one of these. Every minute counts for either filling or draining the reservoir, and you, too, can enjoy a healthier tomorrow.

If life is a house, and better health is on the floor above you, there are six steps that you must climb in order to get there.

To get to a higher level of health, you must step up onto each of the steps. Skip one of these foundational ingredients, and the building will totter, the jigsaw puzzle will have holes in it, the stool will wobble, the cake will fall – you will not stay healthy.

The frustrating part of this is that when we are young we tend to feel healthy, and therefore find it easy to neglect these steps. But it is in the early decades of life that we must lay these foundational habits and structural stabilizers if we want them to help us most effectively in later decades.

Now, as I said, it is never too late to add these steps to our routines, because the human body is amazing in its ability to heal itself, given the proper help. But the sooner the better. Don't wait another day. Do not allow another moment of complacence. Sit down with a pad of paper as you read this book and plan specific steps, including when you will start them, the time of day you will do them, and exactly what each action step will be for improving your health regimen.

This book is not an exhaustive look into any of these essential ingredients to health. Many books have been written on each of these topics, but in these few pages I want to bring them into a cohesive focus to help you implement a lifestyle that balances all of them.

As you read, look for ways you can sharpen your focus in each area. Look for, and take notes on, small changes that you can make – changes that you can stick with – in order to do a better job of refilling the reservoir. Small changes, done consistently will make a big difference.

In a later chapter we will show ways to make these notes practical, achievable, and life-changing!

CHAPTER 3 - Building Block Number One:

Sane Nutrition

There are so many diets, so many contradictory opinions, so many downright dangerous ways to approach nutrition, you could try one each month for the rest of your life- and your life would be much shorter. There is a bit of 'insanity' in the way we look for the magic bullet of nutrition. If I eat 'this' I'll be healthy. If I take 'x' supplement I'll no longer have arthritis, fibromyalgia, lose my hair, and I'll have the energy of a corn syrup-injected 4 year old.

Of course supplement 'x' has a different name – the magic root, berry or leaf from the jungles of Ecuador, Indonesia or inner Mongolia – changes every 2.3 years. Just when the latest multi-level scam is about to pay off for me, the miracle cure supplement changes to a new tree, root, bark, or juice. I often wonder, if God had made a miracle drug to cure all diseases, why would He hide it in the root of a rare tree found only in a specific ten mile stretch of remote, crocodile-infested river bank of jungle? Also, why is it that any particular 'wonder supplement' works for some people, and then does little or nothing for most of the rest of us? Chasing the latest nutritional fad can make a person more than just a little crazy.

Let's try to bring some simplicity and sanity to the topic. How about some common sense and moderation in our diet?

How about we simply eliminate the obvious poisons, minimize the suspicious items, and just enjoy balance in life? So here are four practical aspects to the nutritional component of better health.

First, minimize the things that suck important nutrients from our bodies. Sugary, starchy white grains tends to pull vitamins, minerals and enzymes from our bodies simply to metabolize them, and they resupply our bodies with - nothing. Such processed foods drain our bodies of the ability to rebuild healthy cells and tissues. These types of foods also depress our immune response, leaving us more susceptible to bacteria and viral infections. At the same time, life should not be miserable, so don't make it that way by trying to eliminate all of the 'bad' carbohydrates from your diet at once. But cut down on soda pop, processed flour and sugar. Develop a taste for fruits, vegetables, whole grains. This will leave less room for the junky foods that drain so many nutrients from our bodies. We will feel better, have more energy, be healthier and stronger, and function better.

Second, we benefit by planning our eating along the lines of the nutritional pyramid. While the details of the pyramid vary from year to year, we can still improve our baseline nutrition by thinking along these pyramid guidelines.

1) Eat mostly fresh fruits and vegetables.
2) Eat less grains – and only whole grains. This may require some fine tuning if you are gluten intolerant.
3) Eat less yet proteins – and healthy proteins at that. Shift toward whiter, leaner meats.
4) Eat even less fats – and, you guessed it – aim for the healthy fats. Think unsaturated. Liquid, and less processed fats are better than saturated, processed, hard fats.

5) Finally – eat least of all sweets for deserts. A twinky at the top of the pyramid, once in a while, will not destroy your life. Just keep it in perspective, in control, in balance.

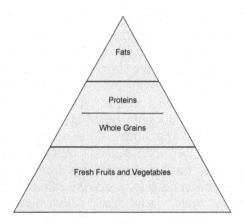

This is the pyramid of nutrition in simple form. Let me warn you – don't stress out over this. It is just a guideline to help us live healthier.

The goal is to shift away from 'dead' processed foods and toward fresh 'live' foods. Live foods are less processed, less cooked, less packaged, less stored. They are foods that are closer to how God made 'em. They look like the way they grew. And they are more complete – that is, the subtle, micronutrients that come along with the vitamins and minerals are still there. These micronutrients are too dilute to be labeled as key food requirements by the governmental testing, but are essential to make vitamins and minerals more readily useable by the cells in our bodies. Whole foods – raw foods – live foods – have these micronutrients packaged right along with the vitamins and minerals, and they are crucial to keeping the reservoir full.

Third, once we have your eating balanced along the lines of the nutritional pyramid, it is still important to supplement. I know, I can hear it now – "But I eat a lot of veggies and fruits! I don't need to supplement."

Let me tell you why I disagree. The foods we eat are not what they used to be. (Don't I sound like an 80 year old, living-in-the-past, shriveled up, old man?) But they are not. One study compared a dinner salad today to one 20 years ago, and found that it takes 12 salads today to provide the nutritional components of one salad back in the good old days! Twelve of them!

The reason? Our fruits and vegetables arrive at our table via a different process than they used to. First, they are grown in soils that are overused, and therefore drained of some of the nutritional components that allow proper 'topping off' of the content in the vegetables that are picked.

Second, because we expect the vegetables and fruits to be ripe when they are sold at the store, they must be harvested before they are ripe. This allows the produce to ripen en route to the store, stashed away in the back of a truck, rather than still attached to the root where it could have been packing away further vitamins and minerals. It's difficult to do this in the back of a truck driving 70 miles each hour across I-70 in the middle of Kansas.

Then we freeze them, store them, expose them to air, process them, cook them and further deplete vitamin content. All of this explains why a good, basic foundation of nutritional supplements is important too. Yes, even if we eat a lot of fresh, raw vegetables.

But once we decide that we are going to supplement, there are still decisions to make – nutritional nuances to navigate.

There are many vitamin suppliers to choose between. How do we know which companies provide what they claim? And does it make a difference? Is a $20 per month product really twice as good as a $10 per month product?

The answer lies in the word 'bioavailability'. You basically get what you pay for in vitamins, and some are more 'bio-available' than others. In fact, the one per day, candy-coated, cheaper vitamins have been shown to simply flow through the digestive system and 90% of each pill is flushed down the drain. Only 10% is actually digested, absorbed and used.

Bioavailable vitamins take into account four factors that the cheaper vitamins ignore.
- The timing at which the supplement dissolves in the digestive tract. Different vitamins are absorbed at different places along the intestinal trail, and if they are available too early or too late, they will not get absorbed.
- Then when they do dissolve, the minerals must be the right size to pass through the intestinal wall. Minerals are basically powdered stone, and must be appropriately sized to make it through the pores in the lining of the gut into the blood stream.
- Once the vitamins and minerals are in the blood, they must have the right ionic makeup to pass through each cell wall and get inside the cells where they do their metabolic work.
- Finally, there is the matter of 'whole foods'. While vitamins have a molecular makeup that can be mapped and copied in a lab, there are micro-nutrients that accompany those vitamins in nature that enable their proper metabolism. Those micro-nutrients are impossible to duplicate in a lab, and can

only be 'packaged' with the vitamin when the vitamins are taken from whole foods.

These four factors are the difference between cheap vitamins and 'natural', or bioavailable vitamins. These factors are why it pays to invest in a better product.

So now the question is, "How do we know if a vitamin is bioavailable or not?" There are many quality products out there, and there are a lot of cheap products. Research can reveal which ones are which, and there are web sites that can help you sort them out. Or you can ask qualified people at quality health food stores for advice.

In our office, we've done some of the research and have partnered with companies that we trust. So look for and stick with a company that is consistent, bio-available, and cost effective.

The next question to answer is what specific vitamin and mineral combination should you take on a regular basis. Whatever high quality vitamin brand you decide to use, start with the basics before spending a lot of money on individual vitamins. There are three basics for the typical adult:

-   A daily multi-vitamin and mineral for the basic raw materials needed for repair and everyday function.
-   Balanced soluble and insoluble fiber for healthy heart, digestive system, and cholesterol control. Soluble fiber is absorbed into your blood stream, and is important for cholesterol control, and certain anti-cancer factors. Insoluble fiber is basically roughage. It stays in your intestines and is important for intestinal cleansing, certain anti-cancer factors, and is what your normal probiotics live on.

- Drink more water. Indeed, if there is a miracle chemical that will improve every aspect of health, it is H2O. In fact, drinking half your weight in ounces of water each day will go a long, long way toward making you healthier all by itself. So if you weigh 160 pounds, drink 80 ounces of water each day. That's about a half a gallon, to which you can add some variety by substituting unsweetened juice or tea for part of it.

These three basics form the infrastructure of nutrition. Your nutritional pyramid will stand strong if these basics are a regular part of your daily routine.

Once these are in place, you may then decide that you have need for additional, condition-specific supplements. But get the infrastructure in place first to ensure proper use of all your supplements. You will absorb them better, and your body will use them smarter.

Some examples of additional nutritional supplements may include:
- Anti-oxidant group for anti-aging, anti-cancer, and immune factors – Omega 3, E, C, etc.
- Joint health supplements - glucosamine
- Brain and nerve maintenance – B complex, E, etc.
- Digestive support – enzymes, or probiotics
- Anti-inflammation – water, D, Omega 3, etc.

This protocol will extend your life, prevent some fearful diseases, add energy to your day, and boost your immune system. Doing it the way I've outlined here will also save you money, both on your supplements and on health care.

28

Wherever you are now with your nutrition, improve it in some way – today. Take a moment right now and write down what you are going to change and when. Make this a priority, because your health and your future depend upon it.

Chapter 4 – Building Block Number 2
The Rest of Your Life

Quantity of rest is important. Quality of rest is just as important. So we have two questions - How much is 'enough', and how do we get 'quality' in our sleep? Research shows that we need 7-9 hours of quality sleep daily to function at our best. In fact, one study showed that getting either too much or too little sleep will impact our health in a number of negative ways – so much so that our life expectancy will suffer! Look at the list of health issues that result from not getting the right amount of quality sleep:

Poor healing,
Buildup of stress,
Weight gain,
Heart disease,
Allergies,
Immunity issues,
Mood swings,
Insulin problems,
Other blood chemistry imbalances,
Higher incidents of accidents,
Learning disabilities,
Poor memory,
--- No wonder poor quality sleep results in a shorter lifespan!

Quality sleep is defined as 4-5 complete sleep cycles in a night. The complete cycle is important for emotional healing, stress management, and physical healing, cell replacement, and organic repairs. All of the stages of a cycle are important, so uninterrupted cycles are a key to quality sleep. It is clear that the 4 complete cycles do not necessarily have to happen consecutively, there can be an awake time between cycles (to use the rest room, for instance), but each individual cycle must be complete to count toward a healthy night's sleep.

So how do we get enough quality sleep?

There are a number of factors that will impact the quality of our sleep, and most of them we can control – at least to some extent. So to ensure high quality sleep, be sure to:

- **Minimize noise** – silence or 'white noise' are best. Background music or TV seem to trigger thought processes that impact sleep cycles in a negative way.
- **Dark is better** than light. A night light, or a hallway light can impact sleep cycles, keeping you from optimum sleep. For some, even the light from a bedside clock can be too much light to allow quality sleep.
- **Stay on schedule**. Sleep is controlled by chemical changes in your brain – chemical levels that are patterned. Going to bed within 15 minutes of the same time each night helps those patterns work with you, rather than fighting your sleep patterns.
- **Stay off your stomach**. Sleeping on your stomach is hard on your low back as well as your neck.
- Whether you sleep on your back or side, **support your neck** more than your head by using either a contour pillow or a rolled up towel under your neck.
- Use **a mattress that supports** firmly, yet allows comfort. Cement is too hard, feathers and 'memory foam' are too soft.

- If you sleep on a water bed, fill the mattress firmly. (Though it doesn't really matter if you use soft water or hard.)
- Be finished with **eating and drinking** at least two hours before bed time. This helps your body slow down, and keeps blood chemistry simple as your brain shifts into sleep mode. As additional benefit, this also helps with weight loss.
- **Gratitude** – reading through a list of things you are thankful for as you go to sleep has a positive impact on sleep cycles.

Another important aspect to rest is taking several 3-minute down times during the day. Turn off the phone, the radio, and the lights, and sit still for three minutes. During this time think uplifting, positive thoughts. Set aside challenges and problems for this short break and let your mind dwell on only the good things in your life.

Proper rest is critical to functioning at a higher level. Implement proper postural support at night, as well as three or four down times daily. Start today, and refill your reservoir in this important way.

Chapter 5 – Building Block Number 3
Exercise Smarter, Not Harder

In my travels to other countries, one of the images that stands out is that there are very few overweight people in third world countries. One reason for this is that people rely on their feet for transportation far more overseas than in the USA. If there is one thing that would make the quickest change in people's energy and overall health it is exercise. Not vigorous, "work till you drop" exercise, but simply moderate exercise, like walking or bike riding, on a regular basis. As in for 30 to 40 minutes. Daily. As in every day.

Exercise is critical to optimizing health. It impacts your health in a surprisingly wide number of ways:

Heart rate, circulation, blood pressure, lung function, joint health, cholesterol levels, digestion, spine, bone strength and calcium uptake, arthritis management, emotional health, improved sleep, muscle tone and balance, lymph drainage – all of these are aspects of health that will improve with regular attention to exercise. None of us can afford to ignore this.

There are five levels of exercise that we must incorporate on a regular basis to function at our peak, and in order to keep our reservoir full of the proper ingredients for health. A balanced amount of each is better than focusing on any one of these items. Let's discuss them each, and then we can find the balance that is best for each one of us.

Spinal stability is first because if we work on the others before we stabilize our spine, we will cause damage rather than improving our health. The best way to begin is to visualize our spinal column as a stack of blocks held upright by guy-wires. Stability starts with making sure the tension or strength of those supportive structures (muscles, tendons and ligaments along the vertebrae) is balanced and equal.

Specific stability of those structures can be evaluated and enhanced by a trained spinal specialist – specifically a chiropractor. Your spinal specialist will prescribe specific balance-enhancing maneuvers for us to do to return balance to your spinal system. Performing your maneuvers will take about 7 minutes to do, and usually you will need to do them twice a day. Total time requirement – about 15 minutes daily – six days a week.

Next is core stability. This is mostly abdominal tone, but also impacts your oblique muscles, as well as your side and back muscles. This toning is best done with a stability exercise ball, in conjunction with a trainer or a video system to teach you how to do these exercises safely and effectively. This system will, require a commitment of about 15 minutes, 4 times weekly. Total time requirement – 15 minutes, every other day.

The third level of exercise is cardio work. This requires us to raise our heart beat for a period of time in order to increase the demand for oxygen in as many of our tissues as possible. We should aim for at least 150 minutes weekly, and our workouts should result in three obvious things. There are detailed heart rate targets that we can figure out and target, but you will know that your workout was intense enough if your heart rate is higher than your resting heart rate, our breathing is deeper – so that you can't talk in a normal voice, and you sweat. All three are good things. All three serve a purpose in improving the level of resources in your reservoir of health.

The key to successful cardio training is to find the type of exercise that you will enjoy. Biking, swimming, running, elliptical machine, skating – anything that you enjoy and that raises your heart rate is fine, and will become fun as you make it a regular routine. Walking can even do the job, but make it count. If you are walking for your cardio workout, "walk big". Make walking count by taking long strides, swing your arms big, add a little bit of a bounce to your steps.

Total time commitment for cardio – 30 minutes, five days a week.

As you add cardio exercise, you will benefit by checking with a physician first. This can give you some specific tips to start with, and make sure you start at a level that is safe and appropriate for each.

The fourth level of exercise, resistance training, will improve joint health, improve muscle tone and elasticity, and improve the calcium uptake into our bones. This is a key aspect to minimizing our susceptibility to osteoporosis – just as important as nutritional calcium intake!

Resistance training can be done with free weights, elastic bands, or weight machines. You don't need to pump iron like a body builder, but you should work the muscles, joints and bones every other day for 15 minutes, using as many major muscle groups and joints as possible.

This area of exercise can pose some risk if you jump into it without proper instruction. So the first step is to get some expert instruction. You can join a gym – they all have trainers who can help you develop a workout routine right for your goals. If you intend to work out at home, visit a gym and pay for one or two quick sessions with a trainer to get started on the right track. Time commitment – 15 minutes, every other day.

Finally, the fifth level of exercise, is balance re-education. Loss of balance is a serious issue as we age. Fully half of geriatric deaths are caused by issues related to falls. Quality of balance deteriorates as we age, due to neurologic compromise that can be halted and reversed with a few simple exercises.

The first one is done by standing in a doorway. Use one finger for stability if you need to at first, but the goal is to stand on one foot for thirty seconds with no touching for support. Once you can do 30 seconds with either foot, you can move on to the next level of exercise.

If you contact our office, we'll be glad to test your accomplishment and then give you the next exercise in sequence.

A complete exercise routine, one that includes all five aspects of a well balanced workout, sounds like a large time commitment. But when we break it down to:
  - Spine stability – 15 minutes daily
  - Core stability – 15 minutes every other day
  - Cardio training – 30 minutes 5 days a week
  - Resistance training – 15 minutes every other day
  - Balance training – about 2 minutes each day.
It doesn't sound so bad. And if we swap some of our TV time for exercise time, we spend less time, and gain a fantastic deposit into our reservoir of health.

Wherever you are now with your exercise routine, you can improve it in some way – today. Make this a priority, because your health, and your future depend upon it.

Regular exercise will be a significant improvement in your reservoir, and in your health! Take a moment right now and write down what you are going to change and when. For now, write it right here on this page. We'll take some time later to make a true goals list for improving the resources in your reservoir of health.

Chapter 6 – Building Block Number 4
Strategic Stress Management

A patient of mine once commented that he had no stress. However, he admitted that he was a carrier. And at first glance he seemed to be right! The world could be falling to pieces around him, and everything seemed to simply roll off his back.

But stress is not a feeling. Nor is it necessarily a difficult circumstance. A certain amount of stress is not even necessarily a bad thing. Stress is anything that happens around you that requires a change from you. A change in routine, a change in temperature, a change in relationships, a change in location. So you can see that stress is unavoidable. In fact, there seems to plenty of stress to go around, particularly as our world changes faster and faster around us.

There are two general categories of stress in life.

1) Acute stress is any sudden, large change in our life situation. A marriage, the death of a loved one, a new job, the loss of a job, moving, a vacation – each of these is an example of an acute stressor, a change in life that results in our body's inner, chemical reaction to that change.
2) Chronic stress is a prolonged, usually subtle, source of change or pressure. A bad relationship, a demanding boss, too much on the schedule with too little buffer or down time, a long-standing illness – these issues of life impact our health in the same way that acute stressors do.

Seeing this partial list of causes of stress response, it is clear that we cannot entirely escape or avoid or consciously decide to not have stress anymore. Too many issues are out of our control, or so pervasive, that it is impossible to eliminate stress completely. But that's okay. We were designed to handle some stress. Our bodies have the ability to deal with a certain level of change. Stress becomes a problem when there is either too much of it, or it stays too long.

The reason these issues are bad for us is that they cause biochemical changes in our physiology that cannot be avoided. Certain chemicals, including adrenaline, epinephrine, cortisol, and over 1000 others, are released into our blood stream when we have these sources of stress present in our life. These chemical changes cannot be controlled by 'being calm'. These changes just happen, and they do affect our health. It may not feel stressful, you may not notice it happening, but stress is occurring in and around you every day.

Some of the results of the chemical changes caused by stress load are subtle, some are obvious:
- ⊙ Visceral fat deposition
- ⊙ Lower thyroid hormones
- ⊙ Lower immunoglobulins
- ⊙ Hormone imbalances
  - Testosterone, estrogen, insulin, etc.
- ⊙ Neurotransmitters
  - Mood changes, tension, depression, memory loss
- ⊙ Low bone density
- ⊙ Blood sugar imbalances
- ⊙ High oxidative stress – rust in the cells
- ⊙ Chronic inflammation

- High cholesterol
- Sleep stress – apnea

When these primary stress responses go on uncorrected in our body, secondary effects begin to show up:
- Anxiety
- Back pain
- Constipation or diarrhea
- Depression
- Anxiety
- Poor sleep
- Fatigue
- Headaches
- High blood pressure
- Insomnia
- Shortness of breath
- Stiff neck
- Upset stomach
- Ulcers
- Weight gain or loss
- Cancer
- Compromised Immune system

You can see how serious this is. Undiminished stress, and the inability to deal with the chemical wash that results from it, causes many serious health problems. Over time, the secondary effects lead to tertiary problems:
- Self Medication
- Substance abuse
- Over Medication – prescription and non-perscription
- Problems with relationships
- Frequent Illnesses
- Loss of work
- Higher health care expenses and debt
- Intergenerational trends of poverty, abuse, etc.
- Increase in general death rate

Some physicians estimate that upwards of 90% of doctor visits are driven by stress response! So, if stress cannot be avoided, what can be done about it? There are actually two practical ways to deal with stress:
- lower the stress load, and
- handle the chemical stew that circulates in our blood when we have stress.

Lowering the stressors in life that drive the chemical changes that wreak such havoc with our health can be as simple as spending time organizing, or as complicated as following a new career path that is more suited to our individual personal makeup. Here are some examples that you can consider.

Simplify your life:
⊙ Un-Clutter your life – one drawer at a time, one room at a time...
⊙ Avoid stressful commitments – stop doing things you just don't like to do: competition, performing, leadership roles, etc.
⊙ Overbooking – learn to say "No, I can't do that." You really don't even need a reason to say no. It's your life!
⊙ Get more advice than you give – It's been said that we were given two ears and one mouth, so we should use them in that ratio. Listen at least twice as much as you talk.
⊙ Organize your life:
⊙ Set clear, small, measurable goals
⊙ Take time every week to think through your priorities, set goals that match them, make plans to accomplish them gradually over time.
⊙ Write your goals in pen – they should be well thought out, and only change with deep thought.

41

⊙ Write your plans in pencil – they will always change. Nothing ever works out just like we plan, and that's okay.

This is obviously just a cursory look at lowering stress levels. Any one of these suggestions has been the topic of entire books. Each of them are worth considering, taking some time to see how they impact your life.

At Delta Health and Wellness Center we offer workshops on each of these topics, and there are similar services in most areas. Call us to enroll in one of our workshops. It is time well spent – or invested in your long term health and happiness.

How about dealing with the impact of the stressors we cannot get rid of? Here is another list of ideas. These ones are designed to burn up those potentially harmful chemicals that are circulating in your blood system.

Manage stress by:
⊙ Exercise burns up the chemicals that used to be burned up while running away from an attacking lion.
⊙ Massage Therapy – there is something about human touch that lowers the levels of those toxic chemicals.
⊙ Having a pet is reported to lower stress. I've had some pets that did just the opposite. Hm.
⊙ Expressing and communicating issues takes issues out of our mind and gets them out where they seem less overwhelming. A friend or a professional counselor can be a great resource.
⊙ Journaling does a similar thing – it gets stressful thoughts out in the light where they cause less chemical damage.
⊙ Thinking right thoughts is essential to maintaining a calm mind. Negative thoughts, and gnawing worries

will come by, but you do not have to let them stay. "They may fly over, but you don't have to let them make a nest in your hair." Take control of where your mind lingers. Find positive things to cogitate on.

⦿ Speak positive words. Break the habit of rehearsing all of the bad things that are around you. Our words matter. They change things. Decide to speak only positive things about yourself, your life and the people around you.

⦿ Laugh! This is the funnest, free-est, bestest thing you can do for yourself. Find out what makes you laugh and deliberately get it in your life every day. It is healing, burns calories, and adds life to your years.

⦿ Being right with God – there is a spiritual aspect to lowering stress. Take the time daily to grow the spiritual aspect of what makes you – you.

As our world changes faster and faster, as science, politics and the world scene force change upon us in an accelerated fashion, stress will be more and more abundant. Learn how to deal with it wisely, and you will be healthier and happier.

Make this a priority in keeping your reservoir of health full. Fill it, plug the holes in the bottom of it. Keep the resources you need to function well available.

Chapter 7 – Building Block Number Five
Spiritually Speaking

The spiritual component of our lives is by far the most important aspect because it is the essence of who we are, and because it is the part that lasts forever. Does it not make sense to spend some time ensuring the health of our spirit, since it is so important? We can invest time and effort in taking proper care of the five physical "super-essential building blocks of better health", ignore this one, and pay a huge price later. I'm convinced that we must deal with this one, no less than nutrition, exercise and rest, in order to function at 100% of our potential.

There are a lot of ways people try to deal with spirituality. I have found that the Bible has – for my money – the best answers to the questions of faith and spiritual health. Of course, the meaning of Bible has been the subject of debate for over 2000 years, so I would like to amaze you and tell you what the Bible says in 4 short sentences. Are you ready?

1. Accept Christ's gift of forgiveness – what He did at the cross cannot be replaced by any other means to get right with God.
2. In the New Testament, when a seeker asked Jesus what the most important thing to do was, he told the man to "love God and love people". Now that sounds simple, until you try to make it practical. Then each of

our personalities, skills, gifts, talents and preferences makes it a bit trickier. A couple biblical passages that might shed some light on what Jesus might have meant are:

a. Zechariah 7:9-10 "This is what the LORD Almighty said: 'Administer true justice; show mercy and compassion to one another. [10] Do not oppress the widow or the fatherless, the foreigner or the poor. Do not plot evil against each other.'

b. Matthew 25:34-40 "Then the King will say to those on his right, 'Come, you who are blessed by my Father; take your inheritance, the kingdom prepared for you since the creation of the world. [35] For I was hungry and you gave me something to eat, I was thirsty and you gave me something to drink, I was a stranger and you invited me in, [36] I needed clothes and you clothed me, I was sick and you looked after me, I was in prison and you came to visit me.' [37] "Then the righteous will answer him, 'Lord, when did we see you hungry and feed you, or thirsty and give you something to drink? [38] When did we see you a stranger and invite you in, or needing clothes and clothe you? [39] When did we see you sick or in prison and go to visit you?' [40] "The King will reply, 'Truly I tell you, whatever you did for one of the least of these brothers and sisters of mine, you did for me.'

3. There are distinct physical benefits to being spiritually healthy. Many verses in both the Old and New Testaments speak to this. Study these for starters: (*I have paraphrased these in a personalized format.*)

45

- His words are life to me, and health/medicine to all my flesh. Pr. 4:22
- A merry heart does good like a medicine. Neh. 8:10, Pr. 17:22
- The lame man shall leap as a hart. Isa. 35:6
- He will recover me, and make me to live. He is ready to save me. Isa. 38:16, 20
- He will renew my strength. He will strengthen and help me. Isa. 40:31, 41:10
- With His stripes I am healed. Isa. 53:5
- He will heal me. Isa. 57: 19
- My light shall break forth as the morning and my health shall spring forth speedily. Isa. 58:8
- He will restore health unto me, and He will heal me of my wounds. Jer. 30:17
- He heals all manner of sickness and all manner of disease. Mt. 4:23
- According to my faith, let it be unto me. Mt. 9:29
- He gives me power and authority to cast out, to heal all manner of sickness and disease. Mt. 10:1, Lk. 9:1
- He heals them. Mt. 12:15, Hebr. 13:8
- As many as touch Him are made perfectly whole. Mt. 14:36
- <u>Greater things than these you will do. John 14:12-14</u>
- **SATURDAY**:   He heals all those who have need of healing. Lk. 9:11
- He is come that I might have life abundantly. Jm. 10:10
- If I ask anything in His name, He will do it. Jn. 14:14

46

- Jesus Christ makes me whole. Acts 9:34
- He does good and heals all that are oppressed of the devil. Acts 10:38
- The law of the Spirit of life in Him has made me free from the law of sin and death. Rom. 8:2
- **SUNDAY:**   If I rightly discern His body, which was broken for me, and judge myself, I'll not be judged, and I'll not be weak, sickly, or die prematurely. 1 Cor. 11:29-31
- He has delivered me from the authority of darkness. Col. 1:13
- By His stripes I was healed. 1 Pet. 2:24
- His divine power has given me all things that pertain to life and godliness through the knowledge of Him. 2 Pet. 1:3

(If you would like a more complete list of such verses, contact me at my office.)

4. Faith. What a misunderstood word! People tend to think it means something like, "Wishing for the best." Or "Hoping your dreams will come true." But faith actually is an action. It means acting on something you know to be true, even when you can't see it, measure it, or feel it. Faith is what makes the rest of the Bible 'work'.

Okay. That is the Bible in four quick statements. Are you amazed? Now I would encourage you to dig in. Get right with God, and begin an amazing journey for the rest of your life.

The spiritual journey of life has three components, all of which we should be aware,

47

- o a beginning,
- o a living, growing aspect, and
- o a reward, or investment aspect.

The birth of our spirit has to do with recognizing that God is perfect, and that we are not. It occurs when we recognize that, due to God's love for us, He provided a way for us to have a brand new beginning with Him. That way is to accept Jesus Christ as our savior, to allow His historic death on the cross, which happened about 2000 years ago, to be the payment for all the mistakes we have made.

The moment we recognize and accept these truths, God does a miracle in our hearts. He takes all the wrong in us, and replaces it with a brand new, perfectly clean heart. That is the spiritual birth. And it is just the beginning! Once we have this new, clean heart we must then begin to care for and feed it.

That brings us to the growth process of our spiritual life. Growing as a spiritual being has a lot in common with growth as a physical being. It requires nutrients, exercise, and protection from things that are bad or dangerous.

Every day we make choices that will either strengthen and grow our spiritual life, or stifle and stunt our spiritual life. Time spent reading the Bible will feed our spirit. Talking with other people about what God is doing in our lives, and finding ways to help other people with their needs (both material and spiritual needs) are both ways to exercise and strengthen our spirits. And learning to know and love God better, learning to love people better, and discovering how God created us to function, are all ways of protecting our growing spirits from falling back into the earthy, selfish ways of our old life.

It takes intention and deliberate effort to make our new spiritual lives grow strong and healthy.

The third aspect of our spiritual lives is the matter of lasting significance. We are each given gift of inconceivable value every day. That gift is the daily supply of 24 hours. It matters little if you are rich, poor, healthy, sick, educated, uneducated, or come from a wealthy family or a poor one. Each one of us gets 24 hours each day to use and invest as we choose.

The important fact is that, once we decide to use any portion of time – a minute, hour, or day – it is gone forever. It is up to us to decide what we trade each minute for, and the choices are limitless. We can trade any given hour for playing golf, for eating, for watching a soap opera, for visiting an aging parent, or for going shopping. We can trade an hour for reading a book, for surfing the web, for time in a Bible study, for a nap, or for putting new shingles on a roof.

The decision is ours. The key to a satisfying, significant life is making wise decisions about what to trade our minutes and hours for. How do we make such a decision?

Some time is required to be spent in certain areas, giving us less choice over how to invest that. Work or school requires about 8 hours a day. Sleep requires another 8. Eating, cleaning, and maintenance require about 4 hours a day. That leaves us with about 4 hours each day of discretionary time. 4 hours to invest or waste each day.

Now there is nothing wrong with recreation and relaxation. In fact it is healthy to spend some time exercising, napping, and relaxing. So if we are wise we will spend an hour a day doing some combination of those activities.

49

The last three hours can go anywhere we want. As far as significant investment of those hours goes – there are two factors that will help us decide what activities are going to have lasting significance. The longer lasting the results will be, and the more the activity benefits other people, the more the time will be spent in a significant way.

Why is this important? Since there really is a spiritual component to our lives, it means that there is life after death. Somehow, the things we do now will affect the way we spend eternity. So if we invest our time wisely now, we will reap good benefits for eternity later.

Spiritual birth, spiritual growth and eternal significance. Good things to keep in mind, to ponder on, and to invest in to help us keep the reservoir full, and live a well rounded, holistically well life.

Chapter 8 – Building Block Number 6
Neural Integrity

While nutrition, rest, proper exercise, stress, and our spiritual life all impact our health, it is also true that, even if all of those factors are in perfect shape, poor nerve function will inhibit 100% health. Because the nerve system controls everything that the body does, a malfunctioning nerve will interfere with health no matter how many vitamins we take, how much we exercise, and how stress free our lives are.

The difference between the Chiropractic philosophy and the medical model is this:

The medical model of living teaches people that symptoms are abnormal and should be controlled as quickly as possible with medication, with surgery, or with whatever will get rid of the discomfort as quickly as possible. According to the medical model of thinking, if you have pain, you are sick. Likewise, if you have no pain, you are – by definition – healthy. And finally the medical model teaches that it is the doctor's responsibility to make the patient healthy.

The Chiropractic model, on the other hand teaches that health is experienced when your body is effectively adapting to the many stresses in life, even if it means you have some aches, pains, or fever in the process of adapting. In fact symptoms can be our friend! Pain alerts us to the fact that we have a problem. A fever helps our body fight off viruses and bacteria. A headache is no fun, but it is telling us that there is something wrong – something that needs correction, whether it is a nutritional need, a misalignment in the spine, or something even more serious like a brain tumor. Finally,

Chiropractic teaches that the patient, not the doctor, is responsible for living a lifestyle that will bring health.

In short, Chiropractic philosophy seeks to remove interference to healing and health. And if we get rid of interference, and give our body what it needs, it will heal. This is the law of returning health, and it works every time. It's just the way we were made.

I have been a Chiropractor since 1980, and since then I have kept up with related topics including science, physiology, anatomy, several advanced adjusting techniques, disability evaluation, and most recently, a great advance in natural health care, the Pro-Adjuster system.

But before we describe something of this incredible development, let me spend some time laying a better foundation for the neural integrity building block of health. Then we will come back to Chiropractic, and the quantum step in the science of spinal health represented by the Pro-Adjuster system.

The brain controls everything our body does. It coordinates muscles, balance, digestion, chemical balances, our immune system, our energy level – EVERYTHING! It does this by sending messages down the spinal cord, out nerve bundles that exit the spine through small holes between the vertebrae, and then along nerve fibers that go to every organ and tissue in the body.

The problem is that the spine, which is designed to protect the spinal cord, also has to move. And what can move, can potentially move out of proper alignment. In this case, the individual bones in the spine can misalign, irritating the nerve bundles. This irritation of the nerves, causes inflammation, and prevents the neurons from accurately sending the messages to and from the brain. This is called Nerve Impingement Syndrome (NIS).

Picture it. A nerve is "pinched", causing inflammation. The tissue that nerve controls is deprived of its coordinating information from the brain, so it malfunctions too. If that tissue is a muscle, the muscle will tighten and get sore. If the tissue is in the stomach, you will have nausea, acid reflux, gas, cramps or vomiting. If the tissue is a part of your immune system, you will end up with more infections and disease than you would if everything were lined up properly. If the tissue is a sensory nerve you will end up with numbness, tingling, pain, or burning sensations. The variety of symptoms is endless, because any tissue will malfunction without proper nerve control.

Knowing what causes these misalignments can help you avoid them. There are 4 general categories of things that will make a spine lose proper motion or alignment.

- **Macro-traumas** – jolts and jars where you know you got knocked around. A car accident, falling down a flight of stairs, or getting tackled by a fullback, are examples of macro-traumas.
- **Micro-traumas** – minor bumps that you shake off. Bumping your head, missing a step, stumbling on a rug. These are minor issues by themselves, but they accumulate, and can add up to NIS later.
- **Asymmetries** – using one side more than the other over time strengthens muscles on one side more than the other. This pulls the vertebrae of the spine out of alignment gradually, leading to NIS.
- **Toxic issues** – either emotional toxins such as stress, or chemical toxins such as over-medicating, alcohol abuse, pollution, or poor diet will have a negative impact on many aspects of health, including spinal misalignment and NIS.

53

Avoid these issues where you can. But when they happen, the job of a Chiropractor is to help you find things that interfere with normal healing and remove those interferences. The Chiropractor does this primarily by evaluating the spine for misalignments, correcting those misalignments and allowing the body to function normally again.

While most people think of Chiropractors as 'back doctors', in truth we are actually nerve doctors. It is an exciting thing to be able to find interference, get rid of it, and help people recover their full potential for health, function and life again.

Nerve health is a foundational ingredient to keeping a full reservoir. Take some time today to schedule regular spinal evaluations and adjustments into your calendar. Once or twice every month may be enough to keep your spine aligned. This is important, so do it now!

These past six chapters discussed six essential areas of life to monitor and maintain in order to rise to your full potential for health, productivity, energy, creativity and life.
Now let's look at some steps to make it practical.

Chapter Nine – The Steps To Change

Pick up your pencil, pull over that sheet of paper and your planner, give yourself about 20 minutes, and let's see how easy it is to change the momentum of your health from a downward spiral, falsely blamed on aging, into an upward climb to 100% of what you were created to be and to do. Ready?

Here are four easy steps.

READY!

Write down the reasons why you know that your reservoir is not as full as it should be. As you look at the trend in your health, you may notice a decrease in energy, creativity, productivity, or general health. You may see that you are getting ill more often with things you never used to be afflicted with. You may see things that you used to get and get over quickly, but now they stay longer in spite of your efforts to get rid of them. These are reminders of why you are ready for some changes. Write them down.

SET!

Now write down an action step for each of the six super-essential building blocks that make up the reservoir of better health:

- Nutrition
- Rest
- Exercise
- Stress Management
- Spiritual
- Neural Integrity

Be sure to work on all six of the building blocks. You can't just pick your favorite two and expect to have a properly filled reservoir. They all work together. They all impact one another. They each play a role in keeping us healthy.

As you decide on which action steps, or goals, to write down, keep a couple of guidelines in mind. Keep each goal 'achievable'. You don't need to rock your entire world off its foundation to make a discernable change in the direction your health will take. Small changes, done consistently will make a difference. Examples?

Nutrition – Get a more bioavailable multiple vitamin and take it daily. Or shift your nutrition toward more live foods and less processed foods.

Exercise – Schedule proper sessions of all five of the levels of exercise into your week. (This kills two birds with one stone. It works for your exercise goal and for part of your stress management plan!)

Rest – Stop eating 2 hours before bed time. Or change to a pillow that supports your neck properly at night.

Stress Management – Get rid of your pet. (Just kidding!) Start journaling 5 minutes daily. Or change your thought habits to more positive ones.

Spiritual – find a non-profit group and volunteer once a week. Or get your Bible out and read it for 15 minutes every day.

Neural Integrity – schedule a monthly maintenance appointment with your Chiropractor. Or change your posture to a more consistently balanced one.

You can use these. But take some time to make sure the six goals are right for you – that they take you another step in the right direction. Next point in the process?

GO!

When you write your six goals, make two copies of them. Then GO find someone to hold you accountable. Hand one copy of your goal list of six goals to this person and have them ask you once a week how you are doing with each of them.

SET!

Yes, 'set' again. The final step is to set a time frame in which to get each goal in place. A goal without a time frame is just a wish, and we all have enough wishes. Goals must have a target date – in writing.

There you go. **Four Steps** to implement the **Six Building Blocks** in order to make the **Rule of Three** work for you to get **100%** out of your **One** life.

Your potential is right there in front of you. It is waiting. The whole world is holding its breath, waiting to see what all you can accomplish. Step Up! Fill up the reservoir. And live well!

Chapter 10 – The Pro-Adjuster

Chiropractic has been around for over 100 years, and has produced some great results. Chiropractic is built on the idea that the brain controls everything that the body does by sending messages through the nerves. Misalignments in the bones of the spine irritate those nerves, causing inflammation and preventing normal nerve transmission to and, from the body. This misalignment problem is called Nerve Impingement Syndrome (NIS), and causes all sorts of problems – simply by interfering with the brain's ability to control the body tissues properly.

The results of NIS depend upon
- Which nerves are irritated,
- What those nerves are supposed to control,
- How much pressure is on those nerves, and
- How long the pressure is left on the nerves.

There is some irony in the fact that while the sophistication and complexity of the nerve system are what make NIS so dangerous, they are also what make Chiropractic care so important. While many people think of Chiropractic care for backaches, headaches, neck pain, and hip and leg pain, there are many other health problems that resolve when NIS is corrected.

Some interesting examples follow.

A patient who came for care only sporadically, arrived in the office and explained that he was experiencing blood in his urine, and was scheduled for kidney surgery. After that adjustment, the bleeding reduced dramatically, and after the second adjustment, it was gone and never came back.

A couple brought their two-year old son in, concerned that he was barely able to crawl at that age. A series of four adjustments over the course of three weeks saw the boy crawling, then standing with the help of furniture, and finally taking his first steps.

I could fill pages upon pages with stories of patients who came to our office, desperate for help with back pain, headaches, and neck pain, often as a last resort, after years of searching for help, scores of tests, multiple medications, injections and even surgery. One after another found the help they needed when they got their spines adjusted, and got rid of Nerve Impingement Syndrome. The body is remarkable in its ability to heal once the interference with nerve communication is removed.

Chiropractic has produced good results for thousands of patients over the years at Delta Chiropractic Center, just like the help found by patients at Chiropractic offices all over the world for the last 110 years.

In the spring of 2004, we were introduced to a break-through technology that brought about a quantum leap from good results to GREAT results in our office.

The Pro-Adjuster protocol for analyzing and correcting Nerve Impingement Syndrome is the cutting edge in technology for Chiropractic and for spine health. Due to a marriage of computer technology, piezoelectric ceramics, and motion analysis, this computer-controlled instrument determines four separate factors of the motion of each vertebra in the spine. The correction of those vertebrae that have improper motion and alignment is then accomplished with an extremely precise series of taps on those vertebrae.

The precision of that series of corrective taps is so quick that muscles don't start a 'guarding' reaction, so the correction is gentle and comfortable. The timing of the taps uses a frequency that matches each individual vertebra's 'resonance frequency', so the vertebra is eased into place rather than being forced into place.

The results of this precision is an adjustment that is:
- **Comfortable** because the patient simply sits in a relaxed posture,
- **Painless** because of the light pressure used,
- **Safe** because there is no twisting or forcing of the vertebrae,
- **Objective** because the analysis and correction is shown immediately on the monitor,
- **Scientific** because of the amazing use of cutting edge technology, and
- **Effective** because of the precision of the correction.

While we have gotten good results with Chiropractic care for over 110 years, now we are seeing Great results. The people who have experienced manual adjustments over the years are getting better faster, staying better longer, holding their adjustments longer, and are overwhelmingly pleased with the results. A couple more examples from the Pro-Adjuster patients?

A woman who had experienced chronic constipation, found it eased from the first adjustment onward.

A woman who had difficult reactions to manual adjustments has found the Pro-Adjuster to be the answer to correcting her NIS with no side affects.

A police officer with asthma has seen his breathing easier, and his asthma checkups much better by the second adjustment.

A man with carpal tunnel syndrome has found relief when even surgery failed to correct his problem.

A pastor's wife has found her TMJ problem resolved.

In the next chapter we will have several testimonials in the words of the patients themselves. But suffice it to say that we are thrilled with the results of Chiropractic as people seek answers to their health problems, and particularly since implementing the Pro-Adjuster protocols.

Chapter 11 - How Long Will It Take?
The Momentum Of Disease

The single most consistent question I get when talking with new patients is, "How long will it take till I feel better?" A fair question, since most of our patients present themselves in our office with significant discomfort. Unfortunately, it's also the one question that can't be answered. There are just too many factors that affect the healing rate.

First, how quickly will we be able to reduce the misalignment? This is determined by:
- How much discomfort the patient has,
- How long the vertebrae have been misaligned,
- How much muscle imbalance there is in the spine,
- How badly misaligned the segment is, and
- How much degeneration there is.

Second, how well will the patient hold the adjustment? This is controlled by:
- How long the vertebrae have been misaligned,
- How much stress the patient has in their life,
- How quickly the inflammation dissipates,
- How much physical activity the patient continues while in the healing stage, and
- How consistently the patient follows the prescribed supportive activities, such as nutritional support, exercises, stress management, and postural awareness.

Third, how quickly will the nerves heal? Once we get the vertebrae realigned and moving more normally, thus removing the nerve irritation, the nerves still need to heal. There are 5 degrees of nerve damage that can occur from Nerve Impingement Syndrome.

- 1st degree nerve damage is found when the nerve is irritated, but as soon as the irritation is removed, the nerve resumes normal function.

- 2nd degree nerve damage occurs when the nerve is 'bruised' by the misalignment, so that when the irritation is removed, it may take hours or days for the nerve to return to normal.

- 3rd degree nerve damage is encountered when the 'bruise' is worse, and therefore takes longer, perhaps days or weeks, to heal after correcting the misalignment and improper motion.

- 4th degree damage is quite serious, and can take months, to a year or longer, to heal.

- 5th degree damage is rare, and occurs when the nerve is killed. Fortunately, peripheral nerves can heal, but only at the rate of about ¼ inch per year. When you consider that some nerve pathways are two feet long, that nerve may never have enough time to heal.

So the expectation of nerve healing is affected, primarily, by how much damage the nerve has sustained. Unfortunately, there are only two ways to tell what degree of damage there is in a nerve. The first is by removing the nerve from the body and examining it under a microscope – this is generally only done as part of an autopsy. The second way is to remove the Nerve Impingement Syndrome and see how long it takes to heal. You can imagine that most people elect to remove NIS and wait for healing, rather than removing the nerve.

The point of all of this is that there is no way to accurately predict how long it will take to feel better. With a good examination, an experienced Chiropractor can develop a feel for how long it may take, based on all of these factors. Generally, symptomatic improvements will be noticeable after three to ten adjustments. But there are those who notice improvements immediately following their first adjustment, and those for whom relief takes months.

One way to get a feel for all of these healing factors is to consider 'The Train Analogy'. Consider your health, and the changes in your health as a large freight train running down a track. This train can be moving in one of two directions – either toward better health, or toward worse health. For this discussion, let's say the train is moving down the track toward worse health, for instance, back pain.

(As a side note, an understanding of what made the train move in the wrong direction can be helpful in keeping it from happening again. The factors that make health shift in the wrong direction are nearly always multiple and complex. It is rare to have one isolated thing cause a loss of health, even for something as focused as back pain. It is important to look at all of the factors, including nutritional habits, stress, spiritual health, exercise, rest and spinal stability.)

For miles (years) of uneventful (and non-symptomatic) track, the underlying problem is building momentum and kinetic energy, heading unnoticed toward the onset of pain. Suddenly, the train crosses a point on the track where the passenger notices that something is wrong (the pain becomes noticeable).

It is at this point, (or perhaps even farther down the track because the passenger thought it would take care of itself, or that pain killers would fix it,) that the passenger asks for help in stopping the problem, so they call the Chiropractor, and say, "My train is running in the wrong direction, (it hurts,) and I want some help!"

The Chiropractor, wanting to help the passenger, steps in front of the train and begins the process of stopping the train and returning it to the proper direction of travel.

It is crucial to understand that the train has built up some measure of speed to get to where it is. Therefore, fixing the problem is not so simple as standing on the track and holding out a hand to stop it. It requires assembling the equipment, slowing the train, stopping the train, reversing the direction of motion, building momentum back up in the right direction, and returning the train first to the point at which symptoms can disappear again, and then continuing the travel back up the track toward real health again.

In the same way, getting rid of symptoms requires finding the problem, slowing the momentum of ill health, stopping that momentum, reversing the process and then rebuilding stability as the body moves back toward real, lasting health.

So, here again is the question. "How long will it take to feel better?"

As you now understand, the answer is, "I don't know."

Typically, it will take 3 to 10 adjustments to notice a difference, but it can happen instantly, and it can take months. It requires:

- **Finding the specific cause** of the problem through a consultation, exam, x-rays, and Pro-Adjuster evaluation,
- **Correcting the problem** by adjustment of the right segments and correcting other lifestyle imbalances,
- **"Holding" the adjustment** long enough for inflammation to dissipate, which depends on the patient's activities, amount of degeneration, stress, nutrition, posture, and ability to stay on their adjustment schedule,
- **Allowing the nerve to heal**, which, of course, depends upon how much nerve damage there is, proper supportive nutrition, and the level of stress in the patient's life.

Your cooperation and compliance with all of our instructions will make a load of difference in how long it takes. Your assistance, by learning all you can about your situation, will help as well. Your patience in the process will make it bearable for you.

Remember there are things you can do to help this process, so do your maneuvers, take the appropriate nutritional supports, attend the patient workshops, watch your posture and sleeping position, and be careful of activities that are stressful to your spine.

We will get there. Chiropractic does work. Your body is amazingly well made, and will mend.

Chapter 12 – Putting It All Together

So, where do we go from here? In the preceding chapters there is information that can transform your life, adding years, energy, creativity, and productivity, as well as decreasing sickness and stress.

But how do you implement? I have three suggestions that can put wheels on these life-changing ideas.

First, get out your calendar and set aside an hour to think through and plan your next steps. During that hour, write down a next action step for each of the building blocks of better health – nutrition, rest, exercise, stress management, spiritual health, and spine health. While you are there:

- Be specific. Make your next action steps clear and measurable
- Be concise. Write a date for when you will start each action step.
- Be proactive. Include time for planning the next action step after these ones.

Second, get an accountability partner. Find someone who will ask you how it is going, who will confront you when you slide, and who understands what you are trying to accomplish. Get them on board with asking you once a week how you are doing with each of your six action steps.

Lastly, get started. Do not wait. The energy you now feel to make a change will fade as you wait. Do it now. Schedule your planning hour now. Call your accountability partner now.

Following are some short stories of patients who have seen some great results from the Pro-Adjuster approach to better health. As you read them, see if you see yourself or perhaps one of your friends or family in their stories.

There is so much life available to us. Share this path to better health with others.

If you have questions, or a story of your own, feel free to e-mail it to me at DrRoost@yahoo.com.

Chapter 13 – Our Patients Speak

Ann M., Lansing
Over the years I had seen the Delta Chiropractic Center sign from Saginaw Highway as I drove to and from work. I finally decided to stop and try to get some help from them. I had suffered with back and shoulder pain, caused by holding the phone with my shoulder at work.

I felt so much better after my adjustments, that I soon became complacent and stopped doing my exercises, and became more and more irregular with my appointments. Gradually the pain started again, and without thinking about it, (I am a pharmacist's assistant) I started taking a prescription ANSAID medication. It helped, but I know it was only like a bandaid. The underlying problem was still there.

This was brought home to me when they took my medication off the market due to dangerous potential side effects (heart attack and death). My symptoms came back strong, I started getting hand and thumb problems, and I finally decided to give Dr. Roost a call and get back under care.

The staff at Delta Chiropractic is very nice, friendly and accommodating. They were able to work around my schedule, which helped a lot, because my life is very busy. When the preliminary exams were finished, Dr. Roost explained about the Pro-Adjuster system. I was a bit skeptical. I was used to manual adjustments, and I didn't see how it could work. Because I trust Dr. Roost, I decided to try it.

It really works! I wish they had come up with this treatment years ago. I still don't fully understand how it works, but I don't have to. I just get to reap the benefits.

I can now turn my head freely, I can move easier, I have gotten the strength and motion back in my hand and thumb, and I have a lot less pain. Most days are pain fee, and I continue to see progress.

Thank you, Dr. Roost!

Vickie N., Lansing
When I was about 15, I hurt my back in a fall. From then on I had problems. I was going to my doctor for the pain, and he would treat only where the sore spot was, and not my whole body. So the treatments never lasted. It affected my life in a variety of ways. Often I was in such pain and muscle spasm that I would not be able to perform simple tasks for days until the muscles relaxed.

On a Friday before a holiday weekend my back "went out" again, and my doctor's office was closed. I went to the Yellow Pages, and, praise God, Delta Chiropractic was open and nearby.

Right from the start, I felt that I was in the hands of a caring, professional. I found that I was even happy with the office personnel. I was soon healthier than I had ever been in the past. I appreciate the fact that Dr. Roost is able to help in many areas of my health care, and it's always profitable to talk with him on a variety of health issues.

Now, since we have switched over to the Pro-Adjuster, I find that my back holds even longer, my pain level has dropped to a new low, and I am experiencing an improved lifestyle.

I am greatly pleased with my results, and constantly "gossip" about how much you have helped me. I recommend Dr. Roost to everyone I know.

Lois R., Delta Township
I have had Chiropractic care in the past, but always dreaded the twisting and crunching of the back adjustment. I put off my adjustments longer than I should have, and suffered from neck pain, arthritis, and shoulder blade pain because of it.

I heard of Dr. Roost from some friends at church, and finally decided to call for help when stress built up and made my neck even more uncomfortable.

When I got to Delta Chiropractic Center the staff was very friendly and professional. The Pro-Adjuster is a great asset, because Dr. Roost doesn't have to do the manual adjustment anymore. He know exactly what is needed, and where, and the adjustment is actually relaxing!

I now have much less neck and shoulder discomfort. I am pleased with the treatments, and recommend Dr. Roost as a great Chiropractor.

Karen H, East Lansing

I had back and neck problems for years and years before coming to Delta Chiropractic. "Problems" for me were more than just discomfort. In fact, it was not uncommon for the pain to keep me from performing normal activities, including playing with my young children. I'd never considered Chiropractic treatment, rather, I had come to believe that the pain was something I'd always have to live with.

In December of 2002, my husband was having severe back pain, and sought and found help from Dr. Roost. I was also in a great amount of pain, but had never taken the opportunity to go to a Chiropractor. Finally my husband told me that I should quit complaining, and make an appointment with Dr. Roost. So, I did.

I had no prior experience with Chiropractic, so I didn't know what to expect. I certainly wasn't expecting such a thorough exam and approach to wellness. Truthfully, I guess I thought a trip to the Chiropractor would consist simply of a 'cracked' back, and little more.

What I found was that Dr. Roost comes from an approach of not just fixing the problem, but working past that toward better health. So, what began as a trip to the Chiropractor to relieve back and neck pain, became a relationship, a way of life.

Dr. Roost gave me rehabilitative maneuvers to perform to support my adjustments. I now continue to see him for 'tune ups', and I am more mindful of how I treat my back. My back and neck problems are gone. Where once I felt like a prisoner to my back and neck pain, now I feel free!

Thank you, Dr. Roost!

Jim W., Lansing

I have been under the care of Dr. Roost for over 20 years now, for treatment of a low back problem. I have an instable ankle that keeps my back from ever really healing. As a former police officer, I had to wear over 20 pounds of gear which had an additional negative effect on my spine. The demands of police work caused extreme pain in my low back, and eventually caused sciatica as well. I was often incapacitated, and normal daily activities, such as getting in and out of a tub, getting dressed, and biking were very difficult.

With Dr. Roost's Chiropractic treatments I have avoided back surgery, stayed on the job, and have regained much of my ability to function. I walk and ride bike over 10 miles at a time.

And since the addition of the Pro-Adjuster, treatments have a more immediate effect on my alignment, and I am able to walk and function even better. I have had no sciatic attacks.

Without the help of Dr. Roost and his pleasant staff, I doubt very much that I would be able to do normal activities needed every day at work or at home. I have and will continue to recommend Dr. Roost to many of my friends!

Brittany W., Holt

I am a fifteen year old in eighth grade. For the past couple of years I have been scared because I found out I have scoliosis, and I don't want to be crooked for the rest of my life. I'd seen other people who have scoliosis, and it just seemed to get worse and worse until they were all bent over sideways. Some of them even had to have surgery, and put metal bars in their backs.

I went to Delta Chiropractic Center, where they told me there was hope for my back. They took x-rays and found that my scoliosis was already 11.5 degrees.

I started doing my exercises, got serious about getting my adjustments on time, and in three months the scoliosis dropped to 5.5 degrees! I was so excited!

I'm going to stay adjusted, do my maneuvers, and go on beating this spine curvature.

Jamie and Fred M., Lansing

My husband and I both began treatment with Dr. Roost over ten years ago for back problems. Over those years we have come to realize that Chiropractic care is much more than simply relief from back pain, however. Keeping our spines functioning well is the foundation of our health care in that it keeps us flexible, and keeps our immune system functioning well.

This is important to us, because as a teacher and a pastor, we are constantly exposed to many germs and other stressors, and staying adjusted keeps us strong and able to function well. We desire to serve God well in our positions in life, and Chiropractic allows us to do this.

I (Jamie) particularly like the Pro-Adjuster. It works well for me, I hold my adjustments better, and it is easy for Dr. Roost to keep me informed on my progress.

I also have a TMJ (Tempero-Mandibular Joint Jaw) problem that used to cause a lot of pain. Dr. Roost has eliminated this with his adjustments. I am able to talk, chew, and even yawn again without pain.

I would be delighted to tell anyone about the help my husband and I receive from Dr. Roost!

Chapter 14 – Essays on Health and Wellness

A) ONION LAYER THEORY of SPINAL RECOVERY

On occasion we come across a frustrating case presentation in the form of a patient who is responding well to our care until, without warning or apparent etiology, a new set of symptoms suddenly appears. The patient is happy and content with their progress until the new pain begins, and then, understandably, they are upset over an ache or pain that they feel that they do not deserve.

The key to understanding this frustrating time is the fact that we deal more with **spinal and nerve function**, and how that function affects your **overall health** – than with simple **symptoms**. Certainly the aspect of health that gets your attention is the level of discomfort, but much more important is the **clear function of the spine and nerve system**. What this means is that we are in the business of correcting the spine, and returning the spine to full function. We are not in the business of eliminating symptoms. Usually the two go hand in hand, but sometimes we have to work through some uncomfortable symptoms in the process of bringing full, normal function to the spine.

It is much like finding a hidden, non-symptomatic tumor in a seemingly healthy patient's body. The process of eliminating that tumor is uncomfortable, perhaps even extremely painful, but it is critical to the long term health of that patient. Leaving the spine at less than proper function – even if it's causing no apparent symptoms – will cause more damage in the long run (in the form of degeneration, and non-symptomatic health problems like decreased immune function, decreased energy, imbalanced body chemistry, etc.) than getting rid of the malfunction.

Another facet to this process is the '**Onion Layer Theory'** of spinal function. It is apparent that when the spine is injured it will heal to the best of its ability, adapt and learn to get along with the residual damage. When the next injury comes along the new trauma is layered on top of the older injury, and adaptation takes place again. The initial injury is not gone, it is just covered up by adaptive responses, scar tissue, and the more recent trauma. This happens time after time over the course of our lives, resulting in layers of old traumas, some more significant than others.

When we begin correcting the spinal malfunctions (Nerve Impingement Syndrome) we must work with the most recent one first. As that one is corrected, the next older one is revealed and we must work on that one, then the next older one, and so on until we 'unlayer' all of these old traumas. Some of these layers come with changing symptoms, while others pass unnoticed as they heal. But each one must be corrected to return the spine and nerve system to full function.

So, **the key** is spinal function. **The challenge** is getting through the old layers of spinal malfunction. **The question** is – is it worth it to you to work toward 100% of what your health should be?

The patient's feelings about "that last adjustment causing the problem" is understandable from their perspective, and quite frustrating – both to the patient and to the doctor. But the fact is that the symptoms are a result of spinal malfunction that has been in their spine for a long time, just covered up by more recent malfunction.

On the encouraging side of the equation, these older layers of spinal malfunction tend to resolve quicker. Not always, but usually, the deeper layers resolve within a few weeks of quality care and consistent patient compliance.

B) Disc Problems and Chiropractic

As many as **50% of the people** you see walking around every day have disc swelling, disc prolapses, disc degeneration, or some other disorder with the discs in their spine. Of these, only about 10% of them have symptoms related to that disc problem. Just the same, a problem with a spinal disc is nothing to take lightly. In fact, people who have had back pain caused by a disc problem should take their condition seriously.

But what about **Chiropractic care** for those who have back pain caused by the disc?

A couple of facts may help to understand the answer to this question.
  1) **Discs can heal** – though slowly – if they are properly cared for.
  2) **Twisting** is the number one stress that injures a disc.

3) Sometimes the only form of twisting that caused the disc damage is the twisting of the **misalignment** of the spine around the disc.

Disc problems can be caused by a single traumatic event such as a fall or heavy lifting, but usually the 'event' is really the 'last straw' after a long period of disc strain. That chronic disc strain was usually caused by a twisted, or misaligned bone, either above or below the disc.

Chiropractic care is designed to gently move the vertebrae back into proper alignment, thus taking the twisting stain off the disc and allowing healing of the disc to continue. The **Pro-Adjuster is the ideal** way to treat such problems, because there is no twisting involved, it is **precise**, it is **gentle**, and it is extremely **safe** and **effective**.

The Pro-Adjuster is a computer-assisted device that analyzes the spine, and then gently, and precisely taps the vertebrae back into better alignment and better, healthier motion.

Flexion-Distraction is another tool that gently eases the pressure on discs, and allows rehydration and healing to occur.

Using Flexion-Distraction, along with the Pro-Adjuster approach to **gently realigning the spine**, the strain is taken off the disc, giving it a chance to **heal faster**, giving **relief** to the patient, and allowing gradual improvement to **strength, motion, flexibility, and stability**. The vertebrae move more easily, the nerves are given room to heal and function, the muscles can relax, and you will feel and function better than you can imagine. All without adding to your medications, without surgery, and without any invasive procedure.

Delta Chiropractic Center, the first and only Pro-Adjuster center in mid-Michigan, can assist you in making your way back to full health, naturally, even if there is disc prolapse, swelling or degeneration.

C) The Delightful Things In My Life:

During a tough time in my life, I was encouraged to sit, think and write out a list of blessings in my life. This was a valuable exercise, and I would encourage you to do the same. The following is a list of things that I came up with on that day, updated occasionally to this form.

Enjoy reading, and envisioning these. Then make a list of your own to relive on occasion. Feel the stress of the day dissipate as you recall the feeling of:

- A rumbling thunderstorm after a hot, muggy summer day.
- The cool breeze after a rumbling thunderstorm after a hot, muggy summer day.
- Coming across some fragile, delicate white wildflowers in an unexpected spot.
- The hope of better days to come.
- Seeing spring flowers come up where I planted bulbs.
- The boat floating on clear water.

- A steady breeze filling the sails and the water trickling along the sides.
- The wind blowing my hand up and down when I reach outside my open car window.
- The loving arms and eyes of my children.
- Forgiveness – given and received.
- The freedom, wind, exertion, and flow of thoughts while on a bike ride.
- The memory of a hike in the mountains.
- The vista and exultation of resting on the peak after a long, exhausting climb.
- A cool drink going down on a hot afternoon.
- Sleep.
- Recognizing that I am in the middle of true worship of the living Creator.
- The enthusiasm for life that shows in my daughter's joyful songs.
- Knowing that I just helped someone in need.
- Writing a paragraph that clearly expresses my thoughts.
- Coming home at the end of a day.

D) How To Survive The Tough Seasons

I used to hope that if I tried to respond to God's word with a soft heart, then maybe I wouldn't require the heat and pressure of refining to eventually become what God meant me to be. Wishful thinking. Unfortunately, I don't know my own heart, and even my best efforts at introspection and growth fail to uncover and deal adequately with the imperfect nature of my heart. I am partially blind, partially subjective, partially stupid, and partially self deceived and immature. And to be honest, I am secretly happy to live with 'good enough'. I confess that at times I am content that I have come far enough.

Suffice it to say, my best efforts will never accomplish all that God desires for me. So, in His love for me, He allows discipline and refining times, tests and trials to come into my life to get me beyond the comfortable rut in which I live. In recent years my family and I have been through a season of trial and testing that has been painful and exhausting, to say the least, and yet has resulted in spiritual growth that keeps us thankful for the path down which God is leading us.

I now believe that times of testing and refining will come to each of us. Every one of us will be lovingly, gently, and persistently pressed out of our own image, and into the image of Christ. The question I ask myself is, "How do we get through these times with the best possible attitude, and with the best possible outcome?" I think there are several ingredients that go into a positive outcome as we walk through trials and tests.

First, we must trust. We must cling to what He says in His word and to His promise that what He is doing in us, and what He is leading us through, are better and more important than either our comfort, or where we were before the test started.

It helps, too, to think of that word 'through'. There is hope in that word alone, for if we are going 'through' something, then there must be another side to it, an end to it. Take courage in knowing that we are going through a season, not settling down to stay.

I have found that it also helps to quietly think through the worst-case scenarios of a current situation. As I think about what is the absolute worst that could happen, (of course trying not to panic while there), I begin to realize that even if my situation did end up there, which is not likely, it still isn't all that bad. People have lived victoriously and productively through much worse. Even if death results, that eventuality is, for the Christian, the greatest gain. And in the mean time, we are in God's hands. We are here for a purpose, planned by God Himself.

Another important factor in facing trials with a positive mindset is to realize that lasting significance is not found in worldly ease, material accumulation, or success here in this life. It truly is not about this world. Yet everything we do here and now will somehow effect how we live through eternity. No matter how difficult it may get, this life is short and eternity is long.

As we react to our circumstances, not only will our actions and attitudes effect our own eternal situation, they will also affect the lives and eternal destinies of those who watch us – our children, our friends, our neighbors, the people behind the cash registers, the people in the video stores, the mailman, the officer who stops you for speeding, the salesman on the phone – we are on a stage, and the audience is paying close attention to whether your faith is an act, or if it's real. The great cloud of witnesses, spoken of in Hebrews chapter11, is made up of normal people who came through similar valleys of testing victoriously. We, too, are being shaped to join that impressive company of examples, passing on the hope of victory to those who follow.

Every word, every decision, every action is an investment either in the here and now, or in eternity. Every person who we touch with our lives is being influenced by our behavior and attitude. C.S. Lewis commented that there is no such thing as a 'mere human', but that every person is in the process of becoming either a glorious, awesome, sanctified being, or a hideous, monstrous, eternally-damned being. And what's more, how we interact with that person is assisting them in that process. What an awesome responsibility!

Then, too, it is important to cling to His word in the midst of trying times. We must feed on it regularly to wash our minds clean from Satan's attempts to discourage us. Regularly thank Him for everything – even for that thing that is so hard to take that you can't imagine any good coming from it. There is always something good that will come of a test. So, either in recognizing that He has some great good in it, or simply out of obedience, decide to thank Him for even the toughest of testings.

Cling to His promises to meet our needs, His promise to never lead us into a temptation which we are unable to overcome, His promise to always be with us, and His promises to lead us to better in the future.

Admittedly, some of these attitudes and mindsets are difficult to hold on to. In fact, our feelings will frequently tell us that it just ain't so. But while feelings lie, His word is always true. He does have a plan for you. He is working out a great thing in you. He does hold an answer – even to this situation that has you so confused and weary. He is faithful.

Someday we will look back at the heat of refining fire and see the purpose. We will see what we held onto in faith, and we will have yet another thing for which to fall to our knees and worship our Lord. We will finally see our God for the perfect, wise, holy God He is, and we will worship. We will see with our eyes what we have clung to in faith, and we will worship. We will walk through the gate, find ourselves home, and we will worship.

E) Investing My Minutes

How old do you think you will live to be? The average for a citizen of the USA is about 77, and for our discussion we will be generous and say you will survive to be 80.

With this in mind, at the age of 16 the average person has - (60 m/hr x 24hr/dy x 7d/wk x 52wk/yr = 524,160 minutes per year x 70 =)
- 36,792,000 minutes left to live (of which you use up 1,440 every day). If you are 40 years old, then you have a few less. But from the age of 16 you only have 3640 Saturday mornings left on which to sleep in, 25,480 nights to complain about what time you have to go to bed, 50,960 more times to brush your teeth.

551,188,000 breaths. 2,207,520,000 heartbeats. You will use the restroom approximately 80,000 times (assuming you drink enough water, and your diet has enough fiber in it). These are things that you have little choice over. Your body will go on running properly, if you take reasonable care of it, whether you want it to or not, until you grow old and die. Some things you cannot decide or control.

However, during those 36,792,000 minutes – excuse me – 36,791,998 now - you will make literally billions of decisions that will affect your life, and the lives of those around you, not only for this life, but also for eternity. Just in driving a car – in moderate traffic you make over 100 decisions every minute as you evaluate speed, traffic volume, lane changes, signs, weather, other people and so on.

Each morning you make dozens of decisions regarding your clothing, your appearance, your schedule, and your food that will affect your day, your mood, your health and so on.

Each day you make decisions about your attitude, your words, your responses to circumstances, the friendships and relationships you will pursue, how much you will read, how many T.V. programs you will watch, what you will read, what you will allow your eyes and ears to pay attention to. These decisions will accumulate and form the kind of life you will lead over the next – uh – 36,791,997 minutes.

Then there are the big decisions: who will you marry, what will you study, what will your career be, where will you live, will you experiment with drugs and alcohol, will you pursue God or not, when will you move out of your parent's home, and so on. While these decisions get all the attention, realistically, these decisions are merely the result of the decisions you made in the moments, days and weeks leading up to the big decisions.

That is why your teachers, your pastors, and your parents spend so much time trying to help you make good decisions when the decisions are small ones. They are not trying to make your life miserable, they simply recognize the importance of these small decisions in forming the large trends of your life. They want the next 36,791,995 minutes to be good and fulfilling and healthy for you. It is important to remember that once a minute is used, it is gone forever, sealed away to lead to the results and consequences that come as a result of the decisions you made in that minute.

In thinking through decisions and the possible ways to use the minutes, hours and days left of our lives, I got thinking about 4 categories – perhaps you've heard of the four men who were entrusted certain resources in the New Testament, and how they used their talents, and the parable of the seed sown on four soils?

Well, in our analogy, we will call these the Four **Time Accounts** - into which we can deposit the parcels of time as we use them. Just as we can deposit money into various banks or financial accounts and expect various returns on our money, we must deposit our minutes into one of these four Time Accounts, and we can expect certain things in return. I'd like to spend some time discussing these Time Accounts, and the implications of our decisions about them. Again, once you use a minute, it is placed into one of these Time accounts permanently. You are then stuck with the returns promised from that Account.

Let's start with an innocent Time Account called **'The Living Account'**. We all spend a significant portion of our minutes living. This category includes things like work, school, shaving, brushing our teeth, eating, and cleaning our rooms, as well as things like sports, reading, watching T.V., dating, having conversations, and other recreational activities. 'Living' activities are good things. They are largely neutral in terms of their spirituality, but they are good in that they are a part of a normal life – a life which God created to include those 'Living' activities.

However, items in the 'Living' Time Account can become bad things at the drop of a hat. They can go from being things that God made as a healthy part of life – to being things that are downright sinful – as quickly as the snap of a finger. The difference is made simply by our attitude. How you think, and what you think about while doing Living Stuff will dictate whether this is time well spent, or time thrown away forever.

Remember that each investment account results in certain returns on our investment. While money in a savings account will result in interest accrued, and gain you more money, Time invested in the Living Account will result in certain results – usually material rewards for diligence in the activity. Work hard, you get paid better and get better jobs. Study hard, you get better grades and perhaps scholarships, and eventually a better job. God designed life to require a significant percentage of our time going into this account. It is up to us to keep the time invested here from slipping over into another – a bad account where the return on our investment will be bad.

This second Time account is called the **Self Account.** This is a place where you will deposit some of your remaining 36,791,991 minutes into activities that are purely selfish – and always sinful. There are things that we do that involve serving no one and no thing other than our own selfish desires. Things done only to make us feel good at the expense of other people and by breaking God's rules for a healthy life. Drugs, drunkenness, improper physical relationships, lust, stealing, cheating, overeating, gossip, lying, watching improper movies or T.V – these are examples of places in the Self Account into which we can, and all too often do, invest our time.

The result? Yes, there are returns on time invested in the Self Account, too. 100% of the time investing in this account will result in broken relationships, bad habits, guilt, shame, heavy negative baggage carried into later life, sin, and left long enough – death. This is a guaranteed return on your investment in the Self Account. Every bit as sure as the law of gravity.

Third, **The Service Account** is a place in which we spend time doing things for God, or for other people to serve God. This is a good account. A happy account. Time placed in this account can have a very good return.

But this is one of the tricky accounts, because, like the Life Account, what you do is not as important as why you do it, or what your attitude is while you are doing it. Many have fallen into the trap of serving and doing just to feel better about themselves. Many have been so busy doing that they forget all about seeking, knowing and loving God. It is easy to do a service for someone just to be thought well of. It is even possible to do good, visible services at the expense of doing things that are higher priorities. This is how pastors, teachers, and other Christian leaders gradually find themselves deep in sin, while serving a good public ministry, only to be found out in their sin later. They have spent time pretending to serve God when they are only serving themselves and emptying their relationship with God, until they too are spiritually empty, weak, and vulnerable to Satan's attacks.

An account that will be rewarded by every person who sees you invest here. Think of what people will think of you when they see you visit old people, help in the nursery at church, or go on a mission trip! Wow! You are special! But with this mindset, you are also deluded.

Bon the other hand, the Service Account can be a good, and a very important place to invest time, too. If our service is humble and motivated by simple love for God and for

91

people, the investments here can be paid back with eternal blessings and rewards.

Life, Self, Service – what's left? **The Seeking Account** is the last of our four accounts. It sounds like a bad thing, but actually it is the best of the four. In fact, it is the key account that controls all of the others, because the Seeking Account is where we deposit time spent seeking God. Building our relationship with God is the most important thing we can possibly do with our time. It is as we invest time in knowing and loving Him that we are able to keep our motives and attitudes right, allowing the Life and Seeking Accounts to accumulate eternal value, and it is what keeps the Self Account in check.

The Seeking Account is what God created you, and me for. Fellowship with Him, knowing Him better and better, learning how to love Him with all your heart, mind, soul, and strength is what you and I were made for. It is what makes us tick. It is the only place where you will find joy, satisfaction, and fulfillment in this life.

The interesting part of this is that it is done not only with reading the Bible, meditating, prayer, worship and other obviously spiritual disciplines, (though certainly they are each important to this account) but you can deposit time here with anything that you deposit in the Life or Serving Accounts if your attitude and motivation are right. For God created us – not just to be so heavenly minded that we are no earthly good, but also to know Him in our recreation, in our work, in our studying, in our serving. He is there in our reading, our playing, our friendships, and in our routines of life, if we will just seek Him there, encounter Him there, include Him in those activities.

The returns on investing time in the Seeking Account are eternal, unimaginable, incredible, unassailable, incorruptible and offer a double benefit. The things we do here that draw us closer to God will not only effect how we spend eternity, but just as importantly, will result in changes in us now that will see us through tough times in this life. Knowing God is the only sure defense against despair, discouragement, fear, loneliness and lack of hope.

An interesting aspect of these Time Accounts is that they are not separated by steel walls like a vault in a bank, but by screens. Because of this, items in one account can bleed over into another. For instance, time spent in school can fit into the Living Account the easiest, but it can leak into the Self Account, Serving Account, or the Seeking Account depending upon what we are thinking while in school. If we take the opportunity to goof off, or let our mind slide into thinking about the good looking girl we just saw in the hall, the time slips into the Self Account, never to be retrieved again. In that case, the time-deposit accrues a return of sin, bad habits, and all the other results from investing in Self. On the other hand, time in school can be seen as an opportunity to learn about God's creation, and how amazing He is. This time goes into the Seeking Account. The time in school can be used as an opportunity to encourage other students, or the teachers, or to prepare yourself for ministry. This time goes into the Serving Account and gains all the returns attached to that account.

So – the lessons from this analogy of Investing?

1) Prioritize your activities. If you don't plan how you will spend your time, your time will tend to be invested in the Self Account, or the Living Account.

2) If you find yourself investing in Self, take your thoughts captive and immediately change your thoughts to something better.
3) Make Seeking God a priority of every day and every activity.
4) Monitor your motives and attitudes to ensure that your Serving and Life activities are being used and invested in quality accounts, and not leaking downward into the Self Account.

F) ...But I've never had back problems before!!!

The human body is an amazing creation – for a number of reasons. One of the incredible aspects to its function is the number of redundant systems, back up resources and peripheral support levels that are designed in to allow us to go on functioning even with accumulated, significant disease, damage, and trauma.

For instance, in keeping our blood sugar levels in balance the body has more than enough cells dedicated to producing insulin that even if a large number of them weaken, burn out or die, the levels remain constant, the body remains healthy, and you and I are able to go on eating a wide variety of foods without thinking twice about it. Eventually, however, if we go on abusing our sugar intake, we pass a point where the body can no longer keep up with the insulin demand, and we could develop a symptomatic case of diabetes.

The same is true for most, if not all, of our body systems. Specifically, I refer to the nerve system. We are born with far more nerves than are strictly necessary for proper function and health. In addition, there are backup communication systems that can assist the nerves in maintaining health; circulation, nerves, hormones and chemistry, and even the meridian system.

Therefore, the human frame can take an incredible amount of trauma, misuse, misalignment, and even nerve interference, and **not become symptomatic** for years and years. **All this while, damage is accruing and degeneration is collecting in the spine.**

	100% Health Level
Health Reservoir	**ST Point**
	FB Point
	Symptom Appearance Point
"Sickness"	

In this graph, a patient will _feel_ healthy as long as the nerve involvement stays between the 100% level and the level of **Symptom Appearance.** Even though there is spinal misalignment and some nerve involvement, and even though their inner function is less than 100%, they may experience **no pain** for years, until they finally accumulate enough nerve irritation (often through some small, innocuous incident) to be 'the last straw' and cause symptoms to appear.

There are two potentially frustrating aspects to this.

1) The symptoms don't disappear until we return the spine, and the involved nerves – not just back to the Symptom Appearance point, but **all the way back to the 'Feeling Better Point"** (FB Point).

2) The other common cause of frustration is that **stabilizing** the situation so that the symptoms don't return as soon as we stop adjustments requires returning the spine and affected nerves **all the way back to the "Stabization Point"** (ST Point) – Not Just To the FB Point!

As you work on your return to health, it can help to keep these points in mind, so that you don't get frustrated and discouraged. **Health is coming. Keep doing your part, and you will get there before you know it!**

G) Take Your Child To A Chiropractor!

We get many questions concerning Chiropractic and spinal adjustments for children. In this article we will discuss the reasons for Chiropractic care for children, the results of spinal adjustments, and some of the ramifications of consistent spinal care for children.

Research over the years since 1985 has shown some amazing facts about 'normal, healthy' newborns. Included in those facts are the following:
- 90% of newborn babies are released from the hospital with Nerve Impingement Syndrome.

- During a normal delivery the infant's spine is compressed with up to 90 pounds of pressure.
- The MD will often use 70-90 pounds of traction and torsion to assist in the delivery of the child.
- 100 pounds of pressure is enough to cause significant tearing of spinal cord nerves and other tissues.
- Spinal misalignments negatively affect the immune system, causing a greater incidence of ear and throat infections, as well as other diseases.
- Spinal misalignments irritate nerves, resulting in a decrease in health and changes in body chemistry and balance, both of with are crucial for proper growth and maturation.
- Children fall over 200 times by the time they are seven years old.

Basic anatomy tell us that the body is composed of over 70 trillion cells, all of which must function in a coordinated fashion for a person to be healthy. It is the brain's job, by means of messages sent through the nerves, to provide control and coordination for all of those cells. That is how the body is designed to function.

Trouble enters the picture when the bones in the spine are jarred or pulled out of their proper alignment. This misalignment irritates the sensitive nerves in the area. The nerves become inflamed and no longer transmit the proper messages to their target cells. This is called Nerve Impingement Syndrome. (NIS)

Remember, the brain controls everything that the body does, so lack of nerve communication can cause literally anything in the body to malfunction. NIS may cause obvious symptoms, like back pain or headaches, but most of the results of NIS are subtle, causing deep yet unnoticed

97

problems, like scoliosis, degeneration of joints, allergies, digestive problems, colic, and more. Many mistakenly wait to take their children for Chiropractic care until NIS has caused serious, and sometimes-irreversible damage. Fortunately, your Chiropractor is highly trained in finding NIS before it causes serious trouble.

But what can cause NIS? That tiny baby hasn't done any excessive lifting, sat in front of a computer too long, or fallen off their bike yet. Well, research has shown that while poor posture, stress, and trauma can cause NIS in adults, it is often innocent seeming things that cause it earlier in life. Sitting or sleeping with the head lolled over, being carried in awkward positions, and as noted above, the birth process itself cause most of the NIS found in infants.

We encourage consistent spinal care for even young children for three reasons:
- To assist in the prevention of long-term problems in the spine itself.
- To maintain clear brain control over the immune system, allowing the body to fight off viruses and bacteria as it was intended to.
- To allow 100% function of 100% of the body, and to allow each child to achieve 100% of their potential.

Just as maintaining healthy teeth requires consistent attention, so does maintaining a healthy spine.

One might ask, "If NIS is so dangerous, why does the condition go so unmarked by the medical profession?" My reply is that nerve irritation caused by NIS is so common, that it is now considered normal. If everybody lost the use of their right arm, and if this went on long enough that nobody remembered any different, might not that be considered normal? A scary thought, yet NIS exists in our children's spines and goes uncorrected for years.

Consider for a moment what could happen if every case of NIS was found and corrected early in life! That is what we are about at Delta Chiropractic Center. We desire to see every person, from age 1 day to 100 years, free of NIS so they have the opportunity to grow and function and live at full potential through their whole life.

Spinal care is as important to your child's future as is brushing their teeth, going to school, or good nutrition. Spinal care for a child is very simple, gentle and effective. The examination usually requires nothing more than the doctor feeling their spine. The adjustment is a light, gradual pressure on the spine – so gentle that many babies sleep through their adjustments.

Children tend to respond well to spinal correction – they heal faster than adults, have less stress, and hold their adjustments better. We have seen kids with asthma, ear infections, colic, torticollis, and many other problems, recover with amazing speed.

Let me encourage you to have your children's spines checked. The importance of a healthy spine is not fully appreciated until you have an unhealthy one. The potential of a child is often undervalued until they blossom with healthy nerve control.

IN CONCLUSION

There is a lot of good information in this book – information gleaned from 30 plus years of education, practice, study and experience. But information alone is useless. It takes action to make any information beneficial. So in conclusion, let me encourage you – no, beg you – to take the time to put this information into action.

Set aside an hour to evaluate, plan, set goals, and implement.

Evaluate your current situation, particularly in light of the train analogy, and the fact that there is momentum to health. Think for a moment. If the momentum you currently have in your health continues, if you keep heading the same direction you have been, what will your health be like in 10 years?

Assume you change nothing in your health habits, and you continue draining your reservoir of better health – the only thing that will change is that your health will continue to get worse, and the momentum toward ill health will grow.

The good news is that it can change for the better. Remember the Law of Healing? If you get rid of interference, and give your body the materials it needs, your health will improve. It is a law.

So change something today. Pick six small goals to reach, six improved habits to incorporate into your life. Find a friend who will gently remind you why you are doing them, and get them into your routine.

Small changes, done consistently, will change your world for the better.

Dedication and Thanks

Many thanks to my wife for her patience and wisdom in helping me hear what I have said through other ears. Thanks, too, to the people who have taught me over the years. May this book repay, in part, the debt I owe them, by passing on better health to others.